What You Can Do to Prevent Fetal Alcohol Syndrome

A Professional's Guide

By Shelia B. Blume, M.D., C.A.C.

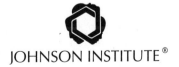

JOHNSON INSTITUTE®

What You Can Do to Prevent Fetal Alcohol Syndrome
A Professional's Guide

Johnson Institute-QVS, Inc.
7205 Ohms Lane
Minneapolis, MN 55439-2159
(612) 831-1630

Library of Congress Cataloging-in-Publication Data

Blume, Sheila B.
    What you can do to prevent fetal alcohol syndrome: a professional's guide / Sheila B. Blume.
        p. cm.
    Includes bibliographical references.
    ISBN 1-56246-043-9
    1. Fetal alcohol syndrome. 2. Fetal alcohol syndrome – Prevention. 3. Fetus – Effect of drugs on. 4. Alcoholism in pregnancy. 5. Pregnant women – Alcohol use. I. Title.
    [DNLM: 1. Fetal Alcohol Syndrome – prevention & control. WQ 211 B658w]
RG629.F4558 1992
618.3'268–dc20
DNLM/DLC
for Library of Congress
                              92-15315
                              CIP

Printed in the United States of America.

Contents

Introduction 1

1. **Ideas About Drinking and Pregnancy** 3
   Ancient Concepts of Drinking and Pregnancy 3
   Modern Rediscovery of Fetal Damage 5

2. **Alcohol: A Teratogen** 7
   The Fetal Alcohol Syndrome (FAS) 7
   Fetal Alcohol Effects (FAE) 11
   Newborn Withdrawal 12
   Effects of Different Maternal Drinking Patterns 12
   Binge Drinking Versus Steady Drinking 12
   Type of Beverage 13
   Mechanisms of Fetal Alcohol Damage 13
   Alcohol and Breast Feeding 17
   Role of Paternal Drinking in Fetal Damage 17

3. **What Is the Risk of Alcohol-Related Birth Defects?** 19
   Epidemiology of FAS/FAE 19
   How Many Women Are at Risk for Producing
   Alcohol-Affected Offspring? RATE 22
   What Is the Risk of FAS/FAE in Women Who Drink
   During Pregnancy? 24
   Other Risk Factors That May Influence FAS/FAE 28

4. **The Child with FAS/FAE** 31
   Understanding the Individual Child 31
   Adolescents and Adults with FAS/FAE 33

iii

5. Preventing FAS/FAE—The Pregnant Woman 35

   Educational Approaches 35
   Screening Women for Alcohol Problems 36
   Educating the Obstetric Patient 39
   Referral to Alcoholism Treatment 39
   Motivation for Treatment 40
   Treatment Needs of Pregnant Alcoholics 40

6. Preventing FAS/FAE—Public Policy 43

   Educating Those Who Need to Know 43
   Professional Education 45
   The Criminalization of Alcohol and Other Drug Use
   in Pregnancy 46
   Policy Recommendations 48

Health Questionnaire 49

**Alternative Health Questionnaire—
"TWEAK" Test** 53

Recommended Readings 55

Introduction

As far as historians can determine, human beings have been manufacturing and consuming alcoholic beverages since before recorded history. Wherever there has been alcohol, there have also been a range of alcohol-related problems, such as intoxication, accidental injury, and alcohol addiction. Thus, throughout history, the teachers, leaders, and governments of societies have sought to warn their citizens about the dangers of alcohol and to establish rules or norms for its safe use. Some of the dangers of alcohol are obvious and are the immediate results of drinking. Therefore, they are seldom disputed. Other dangers, however, are more subtle, more remote in time from the act of drinking, and must be established through more sophisticated scientific study. The damage done to the developing fetus by maternal drinking is in the latter category.

Although alcohol was often believed to have a negative impact on pregnancy, opinions have varied widely over time as to how much alcohol was dangerous, and whether it was alcohol itself, or perhaps other circumstances associated with heavy drinking, that caused harm. Only during the past twenty years has medicine applied the clinical and experimental methods of modern science to the understanding of this most important subject. Although much yet remains to be explained, current knowledge has sketched for us the outlines of a major worldwide problem whose size and importance were unimagined only a generation ago.

The fetal alcohol syndrome (FAS) and fetal alcohol effects (FAE) are now understood to be major causes of fetal and newborn death, mental retardation, birth defects, and learning and behavior problems. These alcohol-related disabilities are also a major drain on our nation's fiscal and health care resources. Even more importantly, FAS and FAE are responsible for immeasurable suffering, family disintegration, and wasted human potential.

Several calculations estimate the prevalence and financial impact of FAS or FAS/FAE on American society. FAS is believed to occur at a

1

rate of approximately one to three per 1,000 live births in the United States. The most conservative of the fiscal impact estimates was published by Drs. Ernest Abel and Robert Sokol in 1991. Using only rates of disability gathered from prospective studies, and omitting the data from American Indian communities where rates of alcohol related defects are often high, these two researchers concluded that for FAS alone, our nation spends $74.6 million per year. About three quarters of this sum is associated with the care of mental retardation. This figure does not include the resources spent on the far larger number of adults and children affected by FAE, nor does it factor in the lost productivity and potential of the victims. Yet the sum is impressive. Preventing a single FAS birth can save society over $150,000.

Since scientific information about drinking and pregnancy has developed only recently, it is important that we learn to apply current knowledge to our techniques of health promotion, education, prenatal care, and alcoholism treatment as quickly as possible. Questions immediately arise that may be difficult or impossible to answer.

- How much can a pregnant woman safely drink without harming her fetus?

- If a woman drinks before she recognizes that she is pregnant, how can she estimate the risk involved?

- Do some patterns of drinking cause more problems than others?

- Does the father's drinking, either before or during the act of conception, have an influence on fetal damage?

- Do other drugs that a pregnant woman might take—caffeine, nicotine, or marijuana—interact with alcohol in specific ways to increase fetal risk?

- What are the best ways to prevent FAS/FAE?

This book is an attempt to present current information in a form applicable to the concerns of educators, counselors, health professionals, and prospective parents. Alcohol is America's favorite drug. We must all be concerned about its effects during pregnancy.

1 Ideas About Drinking and Pregnancy

Ancient Concepts of Drinking and Pregnancy

In the Old Testament (Judges 13:3), a prospective mother is visited by an angel who warns, "Behold thou shalt conceive and bear a son: now drink no wine or strong drink." In 322 B.C., Aristotle observed that drunken women bore abnormal children, an observation repeated in many contexts in the ancient world. In Sparta and Carthage, men and women were prohibited from drinking on their wedding night in order to prevent the conception of a damaged child. Plato also recommended abstinence at the time of conception. How much fact and how much superstition made up these traditional ideas is not clear, yet beliefs about the dangers of drinking during pregnancy persisted throughout history.

In eighteenth century England, the "gin epidemic" afforded an opportunity for clinicians to observe the effect of heavy drinking on childbearing. This historic period, also called the "gin mania," began with the introduction of gin—a potent alcoholic beverage flavored with juniper berries—from Holland.

Early in the eighteenth century, British law was changed to allow the domestic production of distilled liquors from grain. Unlike beer and ale, locally manufactured gin was not subject to taxes. It was a cheap and popular intoxicant, which peaked in popularity between 1715 and 1750 and produced a myriad of social and health problems. Today we are concerned about the proliferation of "crack houses" in our cities. In 1736, there were more than 7,000 "gin houses" in London, or one out of every six houses in the city. Writers of the time observed with alarm that gin-drinking mothers produced children who appeared "weak and sickly; shrivelled and old."

The Royal College of Physicians petitioned the British Parliament to tax gin in order to reverse the epidemic, citing (among other alcohol-related problems) the high rate of perinatal death and the birth of disabled infants. In London, a death rate of 74.5 percent of children christened was reported during this period. Although not all of these deaths were related to alcohol, this and other aspects of the gin epidemic alarmed societal leaders. For example, liquor consumption in England rose from 2 million gallons per year in 1714 to 11 million gallons by 1750. In 1751, a gin tax was levied and gin houses were limited, but the epidemic faded slowly. Interest in drinking and its effects on pregnancy persisted.

Dr. Benjamin Rush, a distinguished American physician who signed the Declaration of Independence and is often called the father of American psychiatry, studied alcohol problems during the late eighteenth and early nineteenth centuries. He considered alcoholism a disease and advised against prescribing alcohol to pregnant women. Dr. Thomas Trotter, a British physician who espoused similar ideas, also warned that drinking during pregnancy led to early miscarriage.

In 1899, Dr. William Sullivan, a medical officer at the Liverpool jail, reported on the perinatal mortality of infants born to 120 "female drunkards." He found the mortality rate more than twice as high as that among the offspring of these women's female relatives who did not drink during pregnancy. Sullivan observed that successive pregnancies in the alcoholic women had poorer survival rates, except that the alcoholic women who abstained during pregnancy (sometimes because of incarceration) gave birth to normal infants, even after having previously given birth to damaged children while drinking. In one of the first scientific studies of this subject, Sullivan concluded that alcohol was toxic to the fetus.

Another early study was a 1905 survey of New York City schoolchildren performed by Dr. T.A. MacNicholl. He reported that 53 percent of 6,624 children of drinking parents could be classified as "dullards," compared to only 10 percent of the children of abstainers.

During the early part of the twentieth century, ideas about drinking and pregnancy changed. Much of this change was due to National Prohibition, the law which forbade the commercial manufacture, importation, or sale of alcoholic beverages in the United States. The law remained in effect from 1920 to 1933. Prohibition's supporters had maintained that alcohol was the root cause of virtually all of the nation's social, economic, and health problems. Because alcohol was initially blamed for nearly everything evil, people viewed ideas about the dangers of alcohol with skepticism after Prohibition's repeal. For example, physicians questioned whether alcohol itself actually caused cirrhosis of the liver, or whether the damage was secondary to malnutrition in the drinking alcoholic. Likewise, the unfavorable outcome of pregnancy, often observed in alcoholic women, was attributed to poor diet, health habits, and hygiene.

On the other hand, theories of eugenics popular during the first decades of the twentieth century, and conclusions based on the limited animal experimentation available at the time led to a different conclusion. Alcohol was regarded by some as a "selective toxin" that would kill off inferior germ cells and allow only the healthy to develop. In this way, drinking before or during pregnancy was seen as something that could actually improve the human race.

Ideas had changed so much by the 1960s, that Dr. Ashley Montague, a distinguished professor of anthropology, could write in his book *Life Before Birth:*

> Unexpectedly, alcohol in the form of beverages, even in immoderate amounts, has no apparent effect on a child before birth. . . . It can now be stated categorically, after hundreds of studies covering many years, that no matter how great the amounts of alcohol taken by the mother—or by the father, for that matter—neither the germ cells nor the development of the child will be affected. . . . An amount of alcohol in the blood that would kill the mother is not enough even to irritate the tissues of the child.

Actually, there had been very little research, and the facts about drinking and pregnancy were still obscure.

Modern Rediscovery of Fetal Damage

 In 1968, a group of French researchers reported on 127 offspring of alcoholic mothers, commenting on their growth deficiencies, facial features, and central nervous system defects. Their paper received little attention until the independent report from a group of researchers at the University of Washington in Seattle, published in 1973, described and named the fetal alcohol syndrome (FAS) as a

5

specific set of birth defects in the offspring of alcoholic mothers. The Washington University report was published in the *Lancet*, a major international journal of medicine. This report was not overlooked. It became the focus of intense scientific scrutiny, with much of the research funded by the newly established National Institute on Alcohol Abuse and Alcoholism of the United States federal government. Shortly afterward, the Research Society on Alcoholism, an organization of concerned scientists, established a Fetal Alcohol Study Group, which continues to meet regularly to establish consensus definitions and share data. Research also began in Canada, Europe, and other parts of the world, where FAS and FAE were also discovered to be major causes of disability.

Strangely enough, many health professionals and public policy makers were dubious about the new information. If alcohol really harmed the fetus, they reasoned, half the people in our country would be damaged. Surely a little drinking couldn't do any harm! Doctors had traditionally recommended alcoholic beverages (in moderation) during pregnancy, as well as beer or ale during breast feeding. Alcohol was looked upon as a mild relaxant. Large doses of alcohol were sometimes used to delay premature labor. Surely, if alcohol were harmful, we would have known it, they reasoned. It took years for standard textbooks to reflect the new thinking.

The Surgeon General's Advisory of 1981 was an important milestone in changing ideas about drinking and pregnancy. The text reads:

> The Surgeon General advises women who are pregnant (or considering pregnancy) not to drink alcoholic beverages and to be aware of the alcoholic content of foods and drugs.

2 Alcohol: A Teratogen

The term "teratogen" derives from the Greek word for monster. It describes any substance or influence that produces birth defects by influencing fetal development. One of the first teratogens to reach public attention was thalidomide, a sedative drug that was widely prescribed around the world, but not approved for general use in the United States. In 1961, clinicians began to notice an increase in births of severely deformed infants, many of whom had imperfectly developed limbs. Clinicians related these deformities to the use of thalidomide early in pregnancy. The drug was withdrawn from use worldwide, but not in time to prevent thousands of individual tragedies. The thalidomide story awakened scientific and public interest in other possible teratogens among the thousands of foods, drugs, and chemicals to which a pregnant women might be exposed. It ushered in an era of more careful monitoring of pharmaceuticals before their approval. Even so, we still know relatively little about the effects of many commonly used substances.

Studies of teratogens have found a wide variety of modes of action. Some have a threshold value: a minimum dose below which no harm is done. The effects of others follow a dose-response continuum, with the amount of damage proportional to the dose, and no safe level of intake. Some, like thalidomide, produce certain kinds of damage only if taken at a very specific time during pregnancy. Others exert their effects throughout gestation. What do we know about alcohol?

The Fetal Alcohol Syndrome (FAS)

The first syndrome recognized to be specific to alcohol as a teratogen was the most severe. FAS is a serious combination of birth defects, seen in the offspring of women who have been heavy drinkers (usually at a rate of six or more drinks per day) throughout pregnancy.

These women are most often the victims of alcoholism. Their risk of producing an infant with FAS increases with subsequent pregnancies, unless they achieve abstinence as part of recovery from their disease.

In order to make a diagnosis of FAS, the following features must be present:

1. **Prenatal and postnatal growth retardation.** Although many FAS infants are born prematurely and would, therefore, be expected to be small, one of the hallmarks of FAS is that the infant is small for gestational age, often below the tenth percentile of expected length, weight, and head circumference, even when corrected for prematurity. In comparative terms, weight and head circumference are generally more affected than length, so that as the infant grows, it often appears thin and malnourished, with a disproportionately small head. While the typical healthy premature infant, although born at low birth weight, exhibits "catch-up" growth to reach normal size, the FAS infant continues to manifest growth retardation after birth and remains small and thin during childhood, in spite of adequate feeding.

2. **Central nervous system dysfunction.** The most obvious manifestations of nervous system damage in FAS are small head circumference, mental retardation, difficulties in balance, and poor coordination. More subtle signs of damage are learning disorders, hyperactivity with reduced attention span, and difficulty in modifying behavior in response to experience.

   Although we don't fully understand the mechanisms that produce this brain damage, it is clear that high levels of blood alcohol during fetal development interfere with the normal growth and orderly development of the central nervous system. In addition, in some cases, major structural abnormalities have been described, such as absence of the corpus callosum, the transverse fibers that connect the left and right cerebral hemispheres.

   Nervous system abnormalities also include the optical and auditory systems (problems in seeing and hearing). FAS children tend to be nearsighted and have small, underdeveloped eyes with short palpebral fissures (the distance from the inner to the outer edge of the eye opening). Poor eye muscle development leads to drooping eye lid (ptosis) or crossed eyes (strabismus) in many cases. Hearing loss has been reported in FAS, and may be related to frequent ear infections due to anatomical abnormality and an inadequate immune system, as well as to nerve damage.

3. **Facial abnormalities.** It was the typical facial defects of the FAS child that led early observers to comment that they all looked like brothers and sisters, or that maternal alcoholism could be read in the face of the child.

The typical face of an FAS-affected child is most distinctive in childhood, but may still be recognizable into adulthood. Its features include a small head with small round eyes, short eye openings (palpebral fissures), and folds of skin on the inner and upper aspect of the eye (epicanthic folds), which, while normal in Orientals, are seen in FAS in other races. The middle portion of the face and nose bridge tend to be flat, and the nose is upturned and short, leading to an elongation of the upper lip. This elongated upper lip has often lost its characteristic central groove, a condition described as flattening of the philtrum. The upper lip vermillion may be thin and the lower jaw small and poorly developed. Teeth often grow abnormally, and the ears may seem large, low-set, and/or deformed.

These characteristics are best understood as results of the slowing of growth of the brain and eye stalks during fetal life. Normal eye growth seems to stimulate the development of the mid-face structures, which are abnormally formed in FAS. Racial and individual differences may make the FAS features difficult to recognize at birth. However, experienced clinicians can often make the diagnosis on sight.

4. **Other birth defects.** Although the three features listed above are needed to establish a diagnosis of FAS, by no means do they exhaust the range of birth defects seen in FAS children. Additional defects range from the mild (birthmarks,

abnormal skin creases on the palms) to the more severe (heart defects, abnormal joints, curvature of the spine, genital and kidney malformations, spinal anomalies, and cleft palate). Any of these may be present in an FAS child and contribute both to early mortality and to lifetime disability.

Figures 1 through 3 illustrate some of the features of FAS.

Figure 1 A B C

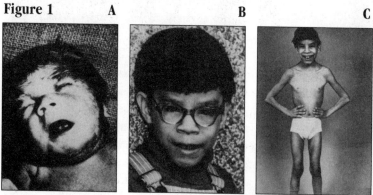

Patient at (a) birth, (b) 5 years, and (c) 8 years.

Reproduced with permission of Ann Pytkowicz Streissguth, Ph.D.

Figure 2 A B C

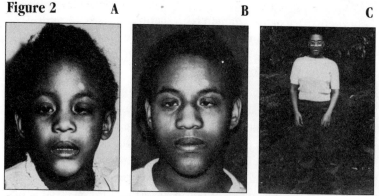

Patient at (a) 3 years, 9 months; and (b, c) 14 years, 2 months.

Reproduced with permission of Ann Pytkowicz Streissguth, Ph.D.

Figure 3   A   B   C

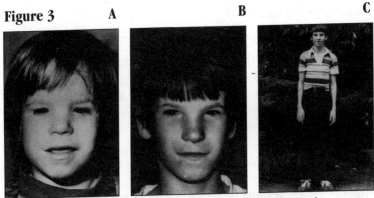

Patient at (a) 2 years, 6 months; and (b,c) 12 years, 2 months.

Reproduced with permission of Ann Pytkowicz Streissguth, Ph.D.

Fetal Alcohol Effects (FAE)

Although the use of the term FAS is specific to a defined group of birth defects that can be diagnosed in an individual child, the term fetal alcohol effects (FAE) has less precision. FAE generally refers to abnormalities presumed to be related to maternal drinking during pregnancy, sometimes expressed as "possible FAE" or "presumed FAE," since low birth weight and other malformations may be due to other causes. In other cases, the term FAE has been used to describe birth defects that satisfy two of the three FAS criteria (for example, central nervous system abnormalities and growth deficiency, but not the facial malformation) and are more certainly a product of maternal drinking. Because more subtle manifestations of FAE, such as small decrements in birth weight, can only be demonstrated in large statistical studies relating pregnancy outcome to maternal alcohol intake, it is often impossible to say with any certainty that a particular isolated abnormality in a child resulted from its mother's drinking. Thus, while a mother may feel that she drank during a previous pregnancy and her child was "O.K.," she may be unaware of subtle deficiencies that put her child at a relative disadvantage. On the other hand, it cannot be said that every child with hyperactivity or learning disability was made so by a mother's drinking during pregnancy.

Newborn Withdrawal

In addition to the growth deficiencies and birth defects that make up FAS and FAE, newborns of mothers who drink heavily until the time of delivery may undergo a syndrome of alcohol withdrawal. Poor muscle tone, jitteriness, and inability to suck adequately interfere with early feeding and responsiveness in these infants. Seizures have also been described. Abnormalities of the electroencephalogram (EEG), which measures variations in the electric currents in the brain, have been found in these infants.

Effects of Different Maternal Drinking Patterns

Although there is no doubt that heavy drinking throughout pregnancy can produce severe birth defects, there is a great deal yet to be learned about the relative risk of varying amounts and patterns of alcohol intake. For some effects, alcohol seems to produce a dose-response continuum of damage. This is probably true for the growth deficiency that leads to decreased birth weight. Other alcohol-related damage is specifically related to the phase of pregnancy during which drinking occurred. Specific structural defects such as heart and joint abnormalities are likely to occur early in pregnancy. However, most women who drink heavily early in pregnancy, but who are able to interrupt their drinking, deliver infants who are not below the tenth percentile in weight. In one study of infants born in Atlanta, Georgia, the offspring of heavy drinkers who had discontinued alcohol use during the second trimester performed better on evaluations of infant behavior at three, fourteen, and thirty days of age than infants of mothers who continued to drink throughout pregnancy. Infants whose mothers abstained throughout pregnancy performed better than either alcohol-exposed group.

Binge Drinking Versus Steady Drinking

Animal experiments indicate that equivalent amounts of alcohol consumed in a binge pattern produce different types and patterns of defects (often more severe), when compared to effects of steady drinking. Evidence on this point from human studies is unclear.

Type of Beverage

Although alcohol in any form, including large amounts of alcohol-containing cough syrup, has been related to fetal damage, there is some evidence that the type of alcoholic beverage consumed may be of some influence. For example, a study of alcohol consumption and birth weight in over 5,000 pregnancies in California found that heavy beer drinking had an especially significant effect in reducing birth weight. The beverage type added to other risk factors such as lower maternal weight and reduced weight gain during pregnancy. Much more research on this subject will be required before the role of beverage type is clarified.

Mechanisms of Fetal Alcohol Damage

Alcohol is an unusual substance. It is, at one and the same time, a food, a drug, and a poison (or toxin). It is a food because it is a source of calories; however, the energy provided by alcohol as a food is generally not accompanied by the vitamins and minerals needed to metabolize nutrients properly. A pregnant woman who derives a significant portion of her daily caloric intake from alcohol is unlikely to be receiving an adequate diet. Although maternal malnutrition alone does not produce FAS, and birth defects similar to FAS can be produced in animals in spite of otherwise adequate nutrition, diet is thought to play a role in the alcohol-related fetal damage observed in clinical cases.

Alcohol is also a psychoactive drug: that is, it is able to alter the drinker's perception, thinking, and feeling. This quality of alcohol accounts for the psychological dependence that is part of the disease of alcoholism. The drug effect of alcohol also influences behavior patterns during pregnancy that increase both fetal and maternal risk. Sleep, exercise, and general hygiene may be disrupted, while personal relationships of heavy drinkers are often stressful. In addition, women who drink heavily are frequently the victims of abuse and violence, whether or not they are pregnant.

Finally, alcohol is a toxin that interferes with the functions of body organs and tissues at many levels. Alcohol is a small molecule that mixes easily in water and passes directly through the human

13

placenta, so that fetal tissues have at least the same alcohol levels as those present in the mother. Furthermore, the fetus has a very limited ability to metabolize alcohol independently and is, therefore, dependent on maternal liver tissue to detoxify this alcohol. Alcoholic women tend to have a higher risk of FAS with each subsequent pregnancy through which they drink. This is probably related in part to increasing liver damage, leading to a reduced capacity to metabolize alcohol. Through this mechanism, the fetus is subjected to higher alcohol levels over longer periods of time.

Exactly how alcohol produces fetal damage is an important question that has concerned many scientists and has led to a variety of animal studies. It is likely that more than one mechanism is involved. Among toxic processes currently under study, the most likely include:

1. Direct toxic effect of alcohol on tissues
2. Toxic effects of acetaldehyde
3. Interference with fetal nutrition
4. Interference with fetal oxygen supply
5. Derangement of the prostaglandin system
6. Interference with growth-signaling chemicals

In examining each of these possibilities, it is important to note that no animal model is exactly comparable to human pregnancy. However, animal experiments are important in establishing that alcohol is an independent cause of birth defects, since nutrition, other drug use, smoking, and a range of unhealthy behaviors can be controlled in a way that is impossible in human experiments. Since various animal species differ both in their ability to metabolize alcohol and in some aspects of fetal development, exact comparisons to levels of human alcohol consumption and types of fetal damage are imperfect. Yet, many important animal findings have led researchers to go back to their FAS human subjects, and, in some cases, have led to the discovery of hitherto unobserved defects—for example, in the kidneys and in the auditory system.

1. **Direct toxic effects of alcohol.** Alcohol has been shown to change the structure and fluidity of the membrane that

surrounds every living cell. Although the ways in which this alters cell function are not well understood, it is quite possible that these changes may make the cells more sticky, in effect interfering with their ability to migrate to the appropriate location during fetal development. Abnormal cell migration is one of the more important findings in the brain tissue of human and animal subjects affected by FAS.

Within the cell, alcohol interferes with a number of normal metabolic processes, including the building of protein from amino acids, a critical part of tissue growth. Although metabolites of alcohol may also be toxic, experiments on animal fetuses nurtured outside of the womb have shown that alcohol alone, separated from its breakdown products, is able to interfere with fetal growth and development.

2. **Acetaldehyde toxicity.** When alcohol is metabolized, it is converted initially to acetaldehyde, a substance that is highly toxic to cells. Normally, the acetaldehyde is immediately metabolized further to less toxic chemical substances. However, a sufficient level of acetaldehyde may find its way into fetal tissues to produce or exacerbate alcohol toxicity. Acetaldehyde from the maternal circulation passes through the placenta to reach the fetus. In addition, the human placenta itself is able to produce small amounts of acetaldehyde from alcohol. The role of this chemical in the genesis of FAS/FAE is not yet clear, but it is very likely to increase alcohol toxicity.

3. **Interference with fetal nutrition.** Malnutrition alone does not cause the characteristic facial abnormalities of FAS, nor do the offspring of malnourished women show the postnatal growth deficiencies that characterize alcohol-related damage. In animal experiments, nutrition is controlled, so that the dietary intake of the alcohol-fed and comparison pregnant animals differs only in the substitution of alcohol for carbohydrate as a proportion of the animal's caloric intake. However, it is possible that part of the mechanism of alcohol-related fetal damage results from interference with

maternal or fetal ability to absorb or utilize essential nutrients. Among these nutrients are thiamine, vitamin B6, folic acid, zinc and other trace metals, glucose, and the amino acids. Experimentation has produced some interesting leads, but no conclusions are possible at present.

4. **Interference with fetal oxygen supply.** Animal experiments and laboratory studies of human umbilical cord blood vessels (tested after birth) point to the possibility that a decrease in oxygen supply may play a role in fetal damage. Blood levels of alcohol reached by moderate to heavy drinkers can cause umbilical cord blood vessels to constrict, decreasing the blood flow and supply of oxygen vital to fetal growth. Research continues to explore the importance of this mechanism to overall fetal harm.

5. **Derangements of the prostaglandin system.** Prostaglandins are chemical components of living cells derived from fatty acid metabolism. They play an important role in modulating metabolic processes within the cell, comparable, at a local level, to the effects of hormones. Prostaglandins are important in every phase of pregnancy and fetal development. Because alcohol is known to increase prostaglandin levels in other tissues, these compounds have been suggested as a possible mechanism for fetal alcohol damage. Drugs, like aspirin, that inhibit the production of prostaglandins have been shown to inhibit some alcohol-related effects. Pre-treatment with aspirin reduced some types of fetal abnormality produced by alcohol in mice, although it did not reduce growth retardation. Further research in prostaglandins will clarify the importance of this mechanism.

6. **Interference with growth signaling chemicals.** Cells grow and divide when signalled to do so by minute amounts of specific chemical substances. This mechanism is important for the repair of damaged tissue, as well as for body growth. Alcohol has been shown to interfere with these processes in several types of cells grown in the laboratory, including central nervous system cells. This suggests another avenue for research on the mechanism of fetal alcohol damage.

Alcohol and Breast Feeding

Just as alcohol travels easily through the placenta to the fetus, alcohol also passes rapidly from the maternal bloodstream into breast milk, and is present in levels roughly equal to the maternal blood alcohol concentration. With larger doses of alcohol, the concentration in breast milk may be somewhat higher than in the maternal blood. The infant readily absorbs this alcohol, which is then distributed throughout the infant's total body water. A case report revealed that a nursing mother's heavy drinking caused pseudo-Cushing's syndrome in a newborn, a condition similar to the effects of overproduction of adrenal cortical hormones.

However, the effects of lesser amounts of alcohol use during breast feeding are far more subtle. Animal experiments in which normal newborns are breast-fed by mothers consuming alcohol have shown retarded brain growth in the presence of normal body growth. A single human study suggests that exposure to alcohol through breast milk causes measurable interference with motor development. Dr. Ruth Little and her colleagues studied 400 infants born to members of a health maintenance organization. Their intellectual and motor development were evaluated at age 12 months. A dose-response relationship was found between the total amount of alcohol consumed by the infant through breast milk and a lower score on an infant psychomotor development scale, although not on an index of mental development. These results were not related to other possible variables such as smoking, drinking, or other drug use during pregnancy. Although the effects found were small, their existence in human infants provides an excellent reason to recommend abstinence from alcohol and other drugs during breast feeding. A recent case report has documented cocaine intoxication symptoms in a 2-week-old baby whose mother took cocaine intravenously while breast feeding. Nothing is known about possible long-term effects, either of alcohol or other drugs consumed through breast milk.

Role of Paternal Drinking in Fetal Damage

One of the most common questions asked about FAS/FAE is "What about the father?" The question is more complicated than it seems.

Since, by definition, FAS/FAE describes damage done by alcohol between the time of conception and birth, drinking by the mother is necessary for its production. However, a pregnant woman living with a partner who is a heavy drinker is likely to find it far more difficult to follow the advice of her obstetrician to avoid alcohol. If she is alcohol dependent and in treatment, the drinking and drug-taking habits of those around her may have a profound effect on her ability to maintain abstinence. Thus, fathers can play multiple roles in preventing FAS/FAE by supporting their spouse's abstinence.

In addition, however, parental alcohol use can affect fetal development by causing damage to the germ cell in either sex (egg or sperm). Such damage could add to the teratogenic effects of alcohol during pregnancy. Although prolonged heavy drinking is known to interfere with sperm production and sexual functioning in both animals and humans, the evidence for a mutagenic effect of alcohol is not clear. Animal experiments have been contradictory. Two brief reports in human populations showed opposite results. In one sample of 377 infants born to members of a health maintenance organization, Drs. Ruth Little and Charles Sing found a correlation between fathers' drinking during the month prior to conception and birth weight, correcting for mothers' drinking, smoking, and other factors that might account for the difference. Another similar study found fathers' smoking, but not fathers' drinking, related to birth weight.

Studies of the influence of paternal alcohol use before conception on older children may be complicated by the effects of growing up with an alcoholic father. For example, a study of 50 children who had grown up with alcoholic father figures found that the children had lower IQ and achievement scales than 50 children of nonalcoholic fathers, even when other possible causative factors were considered statistically. This difference held true whether the fathers were biological or step-fathers, and, therefore, was most likely related to the dysfunctional family environment in which these children were raised.

3 What Is the Risk of Alcohol-Related Birth Defects?

Epidemiology of FAS/FAE

The incidence (number of new cases per year) or the prevalence (number of cases in the population at any one time) of some diseases is known because of reporting systems. Physicians are required to report certain diseases to their state health departments, who monitor these illnesses. For other conditions, data from hospital or clinic diagnoses are collected as the basis of estimates. For FAS and FAE, no general reporting system is in place. Therefore, estimating incidence and prevalence is much more difficult. Physicians often fail to diagnose FAS at the time of birth, even if the newborn is small for gestational age and displays the other features of the syndrome. Even if diagnosed, the code number used to classify FAS cases is not unique for FAS, making retrieval of information more difficult.

Estimating the incidence or the prevalence of FAE from hospital data is even more of a problem, since it is difficult to determine that specific birth defects are alcohol-related at the time of birth without the fully expressed characteristics of FAS. Also, mental retardation and learning and behavior problems may not be evident until well after birth. It is generally accepted that fetal alcohol damage occurs along a continuum from mild to severe. Thus, a single figure for alcohol-related birth defects would be, at best, hard to interpret, and, at worst, misleading. Fetal damage due to alcohol also includes an increase in the rate of miscarriage, an effect that is impossible to monitor in the general population.

Therefore, special methods are needed to develop estimates for the numbers of Americans affected by alcohol-related birth defects. One method is the prospective study, which follows a defined group of women through pregnancy and evaluates their offspring at birth. Some such studies have continued to follow these infants during childhood, so that subtle differences in growth and development can be related to maternal drinking during pregnancy or while breast-feeding. These studies are vital in understanding the relationships between differing quantities and patterns of maternal drinking and effects on the child. However, they are of limited value in estimating incidence and prevalence for the population as a whole.

Other studies are performed retrospectively. That is, they start with data on birth outcome and relate birth weights and birth defects to mothers' estimates of their drinking during pregnancy. Both prospective and retrospective studies take into account a large number of other factors known to affect birth weight and birth defects, such as age, smoking, other drug use, and parity (number of previous births). These studies correct for such factors statistically where appropriate. However, because of their limitations, the two types of studies yield quite different rates of FAS, depending on the populations studied. Racial group or ethnicity also seems to be an important factor in the rates of FAS.

In 1981, the United States Centers for Disease Control (CDC), through its Birth Defects Monitoring Program (BDMP), began to collect data on the race and ethnicity of infants born with 161 types of birth defects from more than 1,200 hospitals across the country. FAS is included in this data system, and the results of monitoring over 4.6 million births between 1981 and 1986 (about 21 percent of all births) have been reported.

The best current FAS estimates provided by the federal agencies involved are approximately one to three cases per 1,000 live births in the United States or about 1,800 to 4,000 infants a year. These rates are based on weighted averages of studies that have varied widely in their findings. Retrospective studies have found much higher rates of FAS than prospective ones (2.9 per 1,000 in retrospective; 1.1 per 1,000 in prospective studies). This may be related to differences in the way women respond to questions about their drinking at different times. For instance, there is some evidence that women tend to underestimate or minimize their intake when the questions are asked during pregnancy. However, other factors such as population differences may be more important.

The CDC's data from its BDMP reporting system reports lower overall rates of FAS, while revealing great differences between the racial and ethnic groups monitored. The rates of FAS reported for the 1981 to 1986 period are shown below in Table 1.

Table 1. Rates of FAS and Down Syndrome*
(in cases per 10,000 total births)

RACE/ETHNICITY	RATE OF FAS	RATE OF DOWN SYNDROME
White	0.9	8.5
Black	6.0	6.5
American Indian (including Alaskan Native)	29.9	6.7
Hispanic	0.8	11.6
Asian	0.3	11.3

*Data from: MMWR 37:17-24, 1988. Leading Major Congenital Malformations Among Minority Groups in the U.S., 1981-1986.

Data on Down Syndrome, another major birth defect associated with mental retardation, are given for comparison. Rates for American Indian infants were 33 times higher and, among Black infants, 6.7 times higher than were rates for white (Caucasian) infants. For American Indians, FAS was the third most common of all major birth defects. For Blacks, it was ninth. Among Hispanic and Asian groups, rates were lower than for whites. Because of marked differences in the incidence of FAS among different American Indian/Alaskan Native tribes, however, these data cannot be used to estimate rates for American Indians and Native Alaskans as a whole. Likewise, because the sample used was not random, the rates for other racial/ethnic groups are not applicable to the country as a whole. However, for comparison purposes, these data are instructive. They are very likely to reflect a combination of variations in genetic susceptibility to fetal alcohol damage and differences in drinking patterns in different groups.

Higher FAS rates have been reported for some American Indian communities, such as the Plains cultural groups. May and his colleagues reported an FAS rate of ten per 1,000 live births among Plains tribes. On the other hand, Southwestern Indian populations, such as the Navajo and Pueblo, have FAS rates similar to those of the country as a whole.

Estimating the incidence or prevalence of FAE is even more difficult. Data from prospective studies varies widely with the definitions and methods used and with the length of follow-up. The best estimates are probably those developed by Dr. Ernest Abel in his book on FAS and FAE. Abel's estimates take into account the differences in the studies reviewed. He estimates that 6,500 to 11,000 infants with FAE are born annually in the United States.

No good estimates are available for the number of miscarriages and/or fetal deaths related to maternal drinking.

How Many Women Are at Risk for Producing Alcohol-Affected Offspring?

To answer this question, we must look at drinking patterns of American women of childbearing age and of populations of pregnant women. There is a great deal of evidence that many women spontaneously reduce their intake of alcohol during pregnancy. This was true even before the "rediscovery" of alcohol's teratogenic effects and the resulting public education. Some women report that they "lose their taste" for alcohol while pregnant. Unfortunately, it is the lighter drinkers who are more likely to find alcohol less appealing. Women who are alcohol dependent are more likely to continue their drinking. Furthermore, some women increase their drinking during pregnancy.

Roughly 34 million American women of childbearing age use alcohol to some extent. National studies of drinking patterns of women aged 18 to 35 reveal that about 78 percent report some drinking within the past 12 months, and about 56 percent report drinking within the past month. A national study comparing pregnant with non-pregnant women found that pregnant women were only half as likely to report any alcohol use as those who were not pregnant.

Of interest is the prevalence of "heavier drinking" (usually defined as an alcohol intake equal to an *average* of two or more drinks per day) among women who are pregnant or just prior to their recognition of pregnancy. This rate has varied widely in different studies, from about 4 percent to 17 percent, and even higher in certain special populations. The heaviest drinkers, *averaging* four drinks per day or more, account for about 2 percent of all pregnant women.

Since women who suffer from alcoholism or report alcohol problems tend to be among the heaviest drinkers and are at risk for giving birth to infants with FAS, rates of alcohol abuse and dependence in obstetric patients are of special interest. Studies of obstetric populations have found that anywhere from 5 percent to 18 percent of pregnant women reported a history of one or more alcohol problems and/or met diagnostic criteria for alcohol abuse or dependence.

In addition, since drinking and other drug use are often correlated in pregnant women and may have an additive effect in producing birth defects, it is of interest to look at current data on other drug use. In 1988, approximately 5.8 percent of American women admitted to some illicit drug use (including non-medical use of prescription drugs) during the month prior to a household survey. Women of childbearing age reported a higher prevalence: 14.1 percent for ages 18 to 28 and 9.6 percent for ages 26 to 34. Among pregnant women, positive urine toxicology screening tests have been reported in 13.1 percent of 335 women in private obstetric care, in 16.3 percent of 380 women in public obstetric care, and in 29.5 percent of 200 women admitted in active labor to an inner-city hospital.

Some researchers have looked at factors associated with continuing to drink during pregnancy in spite of education (and in some cases counseling and/or referral to alcoholism treatment). In a study by Iris Smith and her colleagues in Atlanta, Georgia, 267 Black, disadvantaged women receiving obstetric care reported drinking an average of two drinks or more per week. After health education and/or counseling, 34 percent stopped drinking immediately and remained abstinent for the remainder of their pregnancy. In comparing these women to the women who did not stop drinking, the researchers found that the continuing drinkers were distinguished by higher alcohol tolerance (an indicator of heavy drinking), a longer drinking history, greater probability of a diagnosis of alcohol dependence, a history of previous premature and low-birth weight babies, and drinking with family members. The amount consumed per week and reported use of other drugs did not correlate with continuing to drink. One interesting finding was that women who continued to drink were more likely to report that their mothers were heavy drinkers (9.4 percent versus none of those who stopped). This raises the question of whether these women might themselves have been exposed to alcohol while in the uterus, and whether such exposure might predispose them to alcohol problems. The study also points out the importance of involving family members in the counseling of a pregnant woman who uses alcohol, since the presence of drinking family members will make it harder for her to stop.

What Is the Risk of FAS/FAE in Women Who Drink During Pregnancy?

While the risk of alcohol-related damage to the fetus is zero for a woman who abstains during pregnancy, the risk of fetal damage for one who drinks depends on the quantity and pattern of drinking, phase of pregnancy, and type of fetal damage studied.

Studies of women who were identified as alcohol abusers during pregnancy (a category that would also include alcohol dependent women) have found rates of FAS of 23 to 29 per 1,000. Between 9 percent and 69 percent of these women's infants had some indication (mild or serious) of FAE. However, FAS rates among small groups of pregnant alcoholic women have been reported as high as 40 percent, particularly in economically disadvantaged settings.

As mentioned previously, subsequent pregnancies in drinking alcoholic women have high risk for FAS. One study of an American Indian population found that 25 percent of women who had given birth to one FAS/FAE infant gave birth to others who were alcohol affected. Furthermore, in a review of the literature on FAS, Dr. Ernest Abel looked at the risk for full-blown FAS in siblings of identified FAS cases. Among older siblings, the average FAS rate was 170 per

1,000, while among younger siblings, the rate was 771 per 1,000. The rates of FAE would be expected to be considerably higher.

"Social drinking," defined here as any pattern of alcohol intake that does not meet the criteria for alcohol abuse or dependence, is not generally associated with FAS. However, it is possible for a heavy social drinker to consume enough alcohol to produce the full syndrome.

The question "Is social drinking (or 'light drinking,' or 'moderate drinking') during pregnancy harmless?" has been a subject for discussion since the description of FAS in the early 1970s. I personally took part in a public debate on the subject in New York in 1984, and subsequently published my argument (see Recommended Readings, page 55).

To understand the evidence for fetal damage at social drinking levels, we must consider the difficulties of measuring and describing alcohol intake during pregnancy. There are reasons to believe that self-reports of alcohol intake in general are not very reliable. Subjects in a variety of types of population surveys, including pregnant women, have a tendency to under-report their drinking. The prospective longitudinal study at the University of Washington in Seattle found that self-reports of average alcohol intake in the month prior to recognition of pregnancy (for which the authors established test-retest reliability) was a useful measure. The study's authors found that some fetal effects correlated better with this quantity than with reported alcohol intake in the first five months of pregnancy.

To demonstrate how difficult it is to measure and describe alcohol intake accurately, take a moment or two and try to calculate your own average, daily alcohol consumption. Unless we are non-drinkers, for most of us, this quantity varies from day to day and with the season, holidays, and celebrations. It is quite difficult to estimate one's *average* intake. Furthermore, average figures may be the same for a wide variety of drinking patterns. There is also evidence (as we have seen) that many women spontaneously decrease their alcohol intake during pregnancy, which may complicate recall. In addition, different studies have gathered their self-reported data at different times relative to the onset of pregnancy, a factor that also may affect accuracy of recall. Remember that an *average* intake of two drinks a day does not mean that the research subject drinks two drinks every day.

Very few Americans, male or female, drink daily in uniform quantities. Fourteen drinks a week, consumed by a pregnant woman in one or two sittings, would average two drinks a day but cause a very different type of alcohol exposure for the fetus. Some animal experiments find that a pattern of "binge" drinking (giving the animal a large amount of alcohol at one time) has a greater teratogenic effect than similar quantities given over longer periods. Also, in reporting their data, many researchers use categories such as "two or more drinks a day," which lump the heaviest drinking pregnant women together with some social drinkers.

Genetic factors seem to play a part in any particular fetus's susceptibility to alcohol damage. Thus, levels of intake that are harmless for one fetus may cause harm to another. These factors should be kept in mind in evaluating studies of social drinking in pregnancy.

One documented effect of social drinking is its association with spontaneous miscarriage, especially during the second trimester of pregnancy (months four to six). In a study of 32,000 women participating in a California health care plan, a reported alcohol intake averaging one to two drinks per day was associated with a statistically significant increase in miscarriage, compared to women who averaged less than one drink per day. Those averaging three or more drinks per day had an even higher risk. Another study of miscarriage estimated that a minimum harmful dose was the equivalent of two drinks twice a week. There was a 25 percent rate of miscarriage for women drinking this amount or more compared to 14 percent who drank less, independent of smoking, gestational age, or previous spontaneous abortion.

Social drinking also affects birth weight, birth defects, and postnatal behavior. Much of this evidence comes from Dr. Ann Streissguth and her colleagues at the University of Washington in Seattle, who have conducted a longitudinal study of a largely white, middle and upper-middle class obstetric population and their offspring. This group was drawn from a population of 1,529 women, first interviewed during the fifth month of pregnancy. Their findings have been consistent and included the following:

- 11 percent (6 out of 54) of women who reported one to two ounces of absolute alcohol (two to four drinks) a day gave birth to children with some features of FAS, compared to only 2 percent (2 out of 93) of those women who drank less.

- Social drinkers gave birth to lighter infants. The ingestion of an average of two drinks a day before pregnancy was recognized (and presumably continued through pregnancy) as correlating with a birth weight 91 grams lower than in the offspring of lighter drinkers, independent of smoking. The study's author, interviewed later, was sure that these women were not alcohol abusers. A recent study from the National Institute of Child Health and Human Development confirms this finding. More than 31,600 pregnancies were examined prospectively for birth weight and gestational age. The risk for producing a lower birth weight infant increased substantially when a mother's alcohol intake was one to two drinks per day.

- A study of the behavior of the offspring of women classified according to alcohol use was made shortly after birth. Alcohol use in the social drinkers was associated with measurable differences in newborn behavior.

- The same infants followed at eight months of age continued to show differences. The authors found that the critical level of average alcohol intake prior to recognition of pregnancy, which produced lower scores for mental development and psychomotor development, was between two and four drinks per day.

- At four years of age, 128 of these children were observed in their own homes. The mothers were described as an unusually healthy, well-educated population, whose children were exposed to an enriched environment. The mothers, rated as "moderate" drinkers, drank an average of about one drink per day, with none drinking more than four drinks a day during pregnancy. Their average intake before recognition of pregnancy was between one and a half and two drinks per day. None were problem drinkers.

The four-year-olds of these "moderate" drinkers differed significantly from those of "occasional" drinkers in a variety of measures of attention during mealtime and story time. These children were "less attentive, less compliant with parental commands, and more fidgety during mealtime." During story time, there were differences between boys' and girls' reactions, but both differed from controls. What is the significance of these differences? Perhaps no one can answer that question at this point. However, since animal experiments have shown both increases in activity levels and decreases in learning performance in the offspring of mothers fed alcohol during pregnancy, there is reason to be concerned.

- Analysis of data on over 150 neurobehavioral measures at age seven and a half years continued to show subtle differences between children of women who were social drinkers during pregnancy and those who abstained. These included differences in attention, memory, learning, and problem solving.

In addition to the studies from the Seattle group, five other longitudinal studies, summarized in a review by Dr. Marcia Russell, have looked at the influence of various levels of prenatal alcohol intake on the development of children. These studies involved different populations of women and used different measurements, both of drinking and of outcome. The results have been inconsistent from one study to another. Even so, enough effects have been found to justify concern. Some effects on learning may not be apparent until school age. Thus, the woman who tells her doctor, her family, or herself, "I drank during my first pregnancy, and that child is fine" may not be able to evaluate the truth of her statement.

Other Risk Factors That May Influence FAS/FAE

As mentioned earlier, human populations differ from experimental animal models in the wide range of other factors that influence their pregnancy outcome. Some of these factors have already been discussed. Genetic influences have been described in the literature, but their mechanisms are not understood. For example, in a pair of fraternal twins affected by FAS, one of the infants displayed more alcohol-related damage than the other. Since both infants were exposed to the same amount of alcohol, genetic differences are the most likely explanation for the diversity in disability.

Maternal age seems to be a contributing factor to severity of alcohol-related birth defects—older women who have had previous pregnancies are at greater risk. Malnutrition is another contributing factor. Poverty, with its resulting social and personal stress, makes an additional contribution, either directly or indirectly through increased exposure to drugs and decreased available social support, prenatal care and alcoholism treatment. The use of other drugs is an important contributor to fetal outcome. Table 2, below, summarizes current knowledge about the teratogenic effects of commonly abused drugs.

Table 2. Commonly Reported Teratogenic Effects of Abused Drugs

Specific Fetal Effects	Opiates	Alcohol	Other Sedative-Hypnotic Drugs	Cocaine	Other Stimulants	Hallucinogens	Marijuana	Nicotine
Structural nonspecific growth retardation	X	X	—	X	—	—	X	X
Specific dysmorphic effects	—	X	—	X	—	—	—	—
Behavioral	X	X	X	X	X	X	X	X
Neurobiochemical (abstinence syndrome)	X	X	X	—	—	—	—	—
Increased fetal and perinatal mortality	X	X	—	X	—	—	—	X
Women reporting use in pregnancy (varies with population) Percent	5	>50	<5	≤20	<5	<5	5-34	>50

From Hoegerman et al. 1990
Reproduced with permission of Georgeanne Hoegerman, M.D.

This table is taken from a paper by Dr. Georgeanne Hoegerman and her colleagues at the Medical College of Virginia. Notice that cigarette smoking has been associated with both decreased birth weight and behavioral differences in the newborn. Since most women who are heavy drinkers are also heavy smokers, these effects may be additive.

In addition to the effects summarized in Table 2, an increased incidence of sudden infant death syndrome (SIDS) or neonatal apnea (temporary stoppage of breathing) has been correlated with both prenatal cocaine and nicotine exposure. Heroin dependence during pregnancy has been linked to a range of obstetrical complications and birth defects. On the other hand, women who are maintained on stable doses of methadone, with adequate prenatal care and nutrition, have a much more favorable pregnancy and usually produce infants of normal size and weight. A postnatal withdrawal syndrome is common in their infants, but it can be treated successfully. Although there is some evidence for long-term neurobehavioral abnormalities due to methadone exposure, the research is equivocal. Caffeine has also been studied as a possible risk factor. Research at the cellular level has found that small amounts of caffeine greatly increase the growth-inhibiting effects of alcohol on fetal tissue. While caffeine alone increased cell growth, when added to cells affected by alcohol, it had the opposite effect. Thus, if a pregnant woman drinks coffee to sober herself after drinking alcohol, she may be compounding the damage caused by the alcohol itself.

Other factors do not seem to affect the incidence or severity of FAS/FAE. These include the sex of the fetus and the length of gestation (although prematurity adds risks of other infant damage or disease). Obstetric complications and infections, more common in women who lack adequate prenatal care, often add to newborn ill health and perinatal mortality.

4 The Child with FAS/FAE

Statistical reports of birth weight, neurological testing, and other measurements are important in developing knowledge about drinking and pregnancy. However, the experience of the alcohol-affected child and the family in which this child lives cannot be understood in terms of averages. Each child has a unique set of abilities, disabilities, strengths, and problems. All researchers agree that the *damage done by alcohol occurs on a continuum*. The effects of alcohol range from the very mild to some so severe that life cannot be supported.

Because most FAS infants are born to alcoholic mothers who have been unable to find or profit from adequate treatment, many of these infants are raised in foster homes or given up for adoption. Foster or adoptive parents may not be aware of the prenatal drinking history of the child they are raising. Even if they know the history, it is difficult to assess the full range and severity of fetal alcohol effects at birth, particularly if the infant does not satisfy diagnostic criteria for FAS.

Understanding the Individual Child

In his beautifully written book, *The Broken Cord*, Michael Dorris gives a personal account of his efforts to help his adoptive son, Adam. In raising a child suffering from FAS, Dorris learned only gradually and by painful experience to understand the limitations of Adam's abilities. Since both Dorris and his son are American Indians, the quest for knowledge about Adam's FAS led Dorris to focus in depth on the problem within American Indian communities. Although he found more questions than answers, his book allows us to share the experience of raising such a child.

Typically, Adam was very affectionate and outgoing as a young child. These qualities are often described in FAS. Because Adam seemed so eager and responsive, both his parent and the many

31

teachers and counselors who worked with him felt that he was brighter than he seemed, and that he could function at a much higher level than he did. Each effort was frustrated by another FAS characteristic, Adam's extreme difficulty in learning from experience. Dorris found that other parents raising FAS children and the professionals trying to help them had similar experiences. He writes:

> I remembered Jeaneen's description of children bouncing off the walls of her office in Pine Ridge. "They tend to wander away, need closer than usual supervision. Many caretakers find these children endearing during this period, and their slow development and poor performance is often excused on the basis of their small size. 'Oh, he'll outgrow it,' is a commonly expressed hope at this stage, and developmental delays are often not taken seriously by the family." It was uncanny how her composite results paralleled my own experience, with my folders full of encouragements from Adam's early-grade teachers who maintained, every one, that he was simply young for his age.

Others have observed that teachers, overestimating the ability of FAS children, tend to conclude that they are lazy or stubborn. Because such children are often hyperactive, they may become classroom problems. They often have a poorly developed social sensitivity to other children and find change difficult. In her 1990 Betty Ford lecture, Dr. Ann Streissguth expressed the following opinion: "Now, after 17 years of clinical experience with such patients, it has become all too clear that the accompanying psychopathology is the primary long-term outcome of Fetal Alcohol Syndrome. Management of the behavioral problems is the biggest challenge to their care."

It is, therefore, of particular importance that a child suffering from FAS or presumed FAE undergo a comprehensive evaluation that will allow both parents and professionals to establish realistic educational goals. Training the FAS child for independent self-care and a non-challenging vocational placement may be the maximum that can be accomplished.

Unfortunately, many FAS children have IQ scores just above the level that qualifies them for special community assistance—70 in most jurisdictions. Yet even those who score above 70 are additionally disabled by their hyperactivity, peculiar learning disorders, and inability to adapt. New and improved methods for helping these children are desperately needed.

Adolescents and Adults with FAS/FAE

In April of 1991, Dr. Ann Streissguth and her colleagues published a description of FAS/FAE in adolescents and adults. The study involved 38 males and 23 females aged 12 through 40, all of whom had previously been diagnosed as suffering from FAS or FAE. FAE in these cases described significant birth defects associated with prenatal alcohol consumption that did not have sufficient diagnostic features for an FAS diagnosis. Three quarters of the group were American Indian and 21 percent were white. These subjects continued to show growth retardation into adulthood, with height and head circumference more affected than weight. A quarter of the FAS and half of the FAE patients were not underweight. Adolescent girls reached puberty normally, but some of the boys were delayed slightly. The facial features of FAS became less pronounced with increasing age. Unfortunately, the central nervous system damage persisted. The average IQ of the group was 68, with a range of 20 to 105 (in one FAE patient). The average IQ was lower for the FAS group (66) than the FAE (77).

As a whole, the functional and adaptive level of this group was very limited. Their average grades in reading, spelling, and arithmetic were fourth grade, third grade, and second grade, respectively. Their average level of adaptation was about seven years, although their average chronological age was 17. Only two held regular jobs (as opposed to sheltered workshop employment), and none lived independently.

All of the subjects tested positively for maladaptive behaviors. As Streissguth and her colleagues reported, "The most frequent types of maladaptive behaviors noted were poor concentration and attention, dependency, stubbornness or sullenness, social withdrawal, teasing or bullying, crying or laughing too easily, impulsivity, and periods of high anxiety. In addition, many of the patients were noted to lie, cheat, or steal, to show a lack of consideration, and to exhibit excessive unhappiness. None of the patients were receiving help with mental health problems at the examination."

Most of the subjects lived in unstable family environments with a history of frequent changes of caretaker. Only 3 percent were still with their biological mothers. Recently, alcoholism and serious depression have been reported in several adults with FAS.

This study paints a tragic picture of the long-term disability produced by FAS/FAE. Helping the victims of these disorders must involve a lifelong commitment to their care and protection, which must include managing their behavioral disabilities along with their mental retardation. In 1986, the United States Department of Health and Human Services published a manual with practical guidance for helping adolescents and adults with FAS/FAE. The manual focuses on American Indian communities and is available from the Indian Health Services Office. (See Recommended Readings, page 55.)

The urgency of our need to prevent these birth defects is underlined by the poor prognosis of the affected children. However, the need to establish improved therapeutic systems for the victims of FAS/FAE should not be neglected, and their care, however difficult, must not be abandoned. Sheltered, habilitative environments adequate to their needs must be designed and evaluated. Successful models must then be made accessible to all affected individuals.

5 Preventing FAS/FAE— The Pregnant Woman

Educational Approaches

Education is an obvious first line of FAS prevention. Unless every woman is aware of the risk of alcohol use when planning pregnancy, while pregnant, and during breast feeding, both severe and subtle fetal alcohol damage will persist. Educating men as well as women is also important, since husbands, other family members, and friends interested in the health of mother and child can influence the behavior of the pregnant woman and support her decision to abstain from drinking alcohol.

Research on patterns of alcohol consumption by pregnant women has shown that public education efforts are having some effect. Over the period 1985 to 1988, the percentage of pregnant women reporting alcohol use has dropped steadily (from 32 percent to 20 percent). That is certainly good news. Still, no decline was seen among women under age 25, among those with only a high school education or less, and among smokers. Furthermore, among those who did drink, the average reported number of drinks per month remained the same. Alcohol use in pregnant women remained highest in younger, unmarried, less educated women who also smoked. These groups should be targets for special prevention efforts.

Another way to evaluate the effectiveness of preventive education is by assessing public awareness. Several assessment studies have shown that 50 percent to 90 percent of adults had some awareness that drinking could adversely affect pregnancy. However, few people understood how much alcohol was safe during pregnancy. In a study by Dr. Ruth Little, one third of women believed that an average of more than three drinks a day would not be harmful.

Of course, education alone cannot be expected to accomplish the entire task of prevention. Women who are either psychologically or physically dependent on alcohol (or both) often find it difficult or impossible to stop drinking and stay abstinent in response to information alone. Problem drinkers are usually aware that their drinking is damaging their lives in one way or another, yet the nature of the disease of alcoholism is that the sufferer repeatedly returns to drinking, in spite of resolutions, good intentions, promises, and pledges. Problem drinkers need treatment before they can enter a state of lasting recovery. Therefore, any effort to educate about drinking and pregnancy must contain the message that many women need help to stop drinking and must provide guidance in finding that help.

Screening Women for Alcohol Problems

FAS and FAE prevention will not be effective until all problem-drinking women of childbearing age are identified, treated, and enter a state of recovery. In the United States today, there are approximately 1.8 million women who may be classified as alcohol abusers and an additional 2.8 million who are alcohol dependent. This represents about 5 percent of all adult women. Rates are higher among younger women and decrease markedly in women above the age of 50. According to the estimates of the National Institute on Alcohol Abuse and Alcoholism, the ratio of males to females who abuse or are dependent on alcohol is slightly more than two to one. However, surveys of treatment facilities across the country reveal that the ratio of men to women in alcoholism treatment is more like three or four to one. This shows that *women are underrepresented in treatment.* Women are the "hidden" alcoholics.

If we are serious about preventing FAS/FAE and the many other human and economic costs of alcoholism in women, we must improve our recognition and intervention systems for women.

In recent years, a variety of studies have demonstrated the feasibility of screening for heavy drinking and/or alcohol problems in women within the health care system. For example, Dr. Andrea Halliday and her colleagues at Harvard Medical School employed the simple, four-question CAGE questionnaire to screen women seeking gynecological care. Women who gave one or more positive responses were evaluated for alcohol problems. Twelve percent of the women coming for routine care were suffering from alcohol abuse or dependence, as were 21 percent of those seeking care for premenstrual syndrome. In a study at Johns Hopkins hospital, 12.5 percent of all obstetric and gynecology inpatients were found to be alcoholic after screening. Dr. Marcia Russell and her colleagues demonstrated rates of heavier drinking among obstetric outpatients of about 10 percent, while gynecology patients had even higher rates.

The following questionnaire, developed at Boston City Hospital for obstetric populations, yields a straightforward estimate of alcohol intake.

1. How many times a week do you drink beer?
2. How many beers do you have at one time?
3. Do you ever drink more?
4. How many times a week do you drink wine?
5. How many glasses of wine do you have at one time?
6. Do you ever drink more?
7. How many times a week do you drink liquor?
8. How many drinks do you have at one time?
9. Do you ever drink more?
10. Has your drinking changed during the past year?

From these questions, an average alcohol intake can be calculated. Then, staff can perform an intervention for respondees who have indicated that they are drinking at higher risk ("heavier") levels (for example, at an average of two drinks a day or more) or who indicate a pattern of binge drinking.

The four CAGE questions, developed by Dr. John Ewing and colleagues, can also serve as a good screening tool. The CAGE questions are as follows:

1. **C:** Have you ever felt you ought to **CUT** down on your drinking?
2. **A:** Have people **ANNOYED** you by criticizing your drinking?
3. **G:** Have you ever felt bad or **GUILTY** about your drinking?

4. **E:** Have you ever had a drink first thing in the morning to steady your nerves or get rid of a hangover? (**EYE-OPENER.**)

A third screening tool is the T-ACE, which was developed by Dr. Robert Sokol and his colleagues at Wayne State University. Its questions are as follows:

1. **T:** How many drinks does it take to make you feel high? TOLERANCE (More than two scores two points.)

2. **A:** Have people **ANNOYED** you by criticizing your drinking? (A positive response scores one point.)

3. **C:** Have you felt you ought to **CUT DOWN** on your drinking? (A positive response scores one point.)

4. **E:** Have you ever had a drink first thing in the morning to steady your nerves or get rid of a hangover (**EYE-OPENER**)? (A positive response scores one point.)

A score of two or more indicates high-risk drinking.

A fourth screening approach is the Health Questionnaire designed by Dr. Marcia Russell especially for recognizing alcohol and drug problems in women. Women were found to answer these questions more honestly in a written self-test given in the doctor's waiting room than when asked them by a health professional. Dr. Russell's Health Questionnaire may be found on page 49.

Recently, Dr. Russell developed and tested a simple five-item questionnaire to screen women in obstetric care. It is called the "TWEAK" Questionnaire (see page 53).

Routine blood tests have also been helpful in identifying alcoholic women. For example, blood tests showed that two-thirds of a group of Swedish female alcoholism outpatients—free of physical complications—had larger-sized red blood cells (mean corpuscular volume—MCV) and/or elevated liver functioning (gammaglutamyl transferee—GGT). Again, with a group of problem-drinking obstetric patients from Finland, positive scores on these same tests were sensitive to drinking levels and predicted alcohol-related birth defects.

No matter what type of screening we use for alcohol problems, we need to follow up any positive results with thorough assessment and careful diagnosis.

Educating the Obstetric Patient

Both education about FAS/FAE and screening for alcohol problems in obstetric care should be ongoing. Simply giving the patient a pamphlet or instruction sheet is not sufficient. She should have the opportunity to discuss questions with a doctor, nurse, or health educator at any time during her pregnancy. Most important, when information about FAS/FAE is presented, a health professional should ask the patient about her present drinking, her plans to achieve abstinence, and whether she feels doing so may be a problem for her or for those she lives with. A consultation with family members might be helpful. At every obstetric visit, health professionals should ask patients about drinking and, if necessary, take steps to intervene.

Health care professionals can suggest strategies that the non-dependent woman can use as substitutes for drinking alcoholic beverages. Professionals can encourage patients to think about new ways to handle tension, boredom, anxiety, and other feelings—for example, talking with a friend, taking a walk, or engaging in some other appropriate exercise, or practicing relaxation or meditation.

Another task of education is to evaluate screening results with the understanding that problem drinkers often deny the severity of their problems and the quantity of their drinking. Therefore, do not let a negative test result prevent you from being alert to signs of a possible problem, from repeating a patient's screening at a later time, or from obtaining information from a patient's family members if indicated.

Referral to Alcoholism Treatment

When the obstetric team discovers a patient who is suffering from significant alcohol problems, the team needs to make every effort to refer her to treatment and to see that she completes the referral and becomes actively engaged in the recovery process. If a patient denies that a problem exists or resists referral, take full advantage of other available family members to help in the intervention process. Family members, too, should be referred for counseling and to Al-Anon Family Groups (a 12-step self-help program for the significant others of alcoholics).

Motivation for Treatment

In most cases, pregnancy enhances women's motivation and cooperation in treatment once they have become involved in the process. The desire to have a healthy child is universal. Almost all others in treatment with the pregnant patient are supportive and eager to help. Some pregnant alcoholics will do well in a combination of outpatient care and Alcoholics Anonymous. If there is any doubt about the patient's ability to maintain abstinence as an outpatient, she may need inpatient care or the assistance of a halfway house. A relapse for a pregnant woman has more serious potential than a relapse in any other female patient. If there is a choice, beginning treatment in an intensive, medically supervised, inpatient setting is the best strategy for the pregnant alcoholic. She can then be referred to an outpatient or residential setting according to her individual need.

Several barriers impede women's access to needed care. Many women lack insurance or are unable to access adequate child care for their other children. Recently, limited federal and state funds have been made available for communities to establish special chemical dependence programs for women, including pregnant women, which welcome their children into residential care along with them. These programs teach parenting skills along with other treatment. So far, only a small number of such programs are operating. However, facilities of this type can fill a desperate need in the treatment of the pregnant alcoholic and in preventing FAS/FAE.

Treatment Needs of Pregnant Alcoholics

In addition to the needs mentioned above, the pregnant alcoholic has special requirements for diet, exercise, rest, and obstetric care. The need for obstetric care has sometimes discouraged alcoholism programs from accepting pregnant women, fearing that they may give birth while in the program and subject the program to lawsuits and other liability. To my knowledge, there has never been a lawsuit blaming an alcoholism treatment program for birth defects in the offspring of an alcoholic patient. Fears of such litigation are often expressions of a program's lack of confidence in dealing with a pregnant patient, yet such patients are not really difficult to handle.

Every alcoholism program should have arrangements for the medical care of its patients. Obstetric care is merely an extension of this system.

In some settings, the obstetric care service itself has provided alcoholism counseling to its drinking patients, recognizing that they would be more likely to attend and follow through with a facility known to them than complete a referral to another clinic. This in-program treatment may be effective, but it must be sure to avoid focusing only on the period of pregnancy without offering a long-term support system. The alcoholic woman who relapses after childbirth may start out with a normal infant, but will have serious problems in providing adequate mothering. Therefore, counseling services within obstetric practices will be most effective if they gradually introduce the pregnant patient and her family to sources of long-term professional follow-up, as well as to community self-help groups such as Alcoholics Anonymous or Women for Sobriety.

6 Preventing FAS/FAE— Public Policy

Educating Those Who Need to Know

The role of public education in the prevention of FAS/FAE has been discussed in other sections of this book (see pages 35-36—Educational Approaches). However, there are aspects of preventive education that have engendered controversy in the public policy arena.

The first of these disputes began in the late 1970s with the proposal to require health warning labels on alcoholic beverage containers. The beverage industry successfully fought this proposal for more than ten years before Congress finally passed a warning label bill. The required wording of the label mentioned fetal damage along with other health consequences. Proponents of health warnings consider the present labels an important first step, but are pressing for improvements. Research conducted into the effectiveness of cigarette warning labels found that information was best presented in a rotating series of labels, each presenting a single health consequence rather than a list of unrelated facts. Alcoholic beverages should also be required to carry a rotating series of messages. Furthermore, the label requirements should be strengthened to improve the legibility of the text and to display it more prominently.

Prior to the introduction of warning labels on alcoholic beverage containers, some jurisdictions required that health warning posters related to drinking and pregnancy be displayed wherever alcoholic beverages were sold. New York City adopted the first warning poster legislation in 1984 and was followed by a number of other cities, states, and localities. Alcohol industry lobbyists have argued, in opposition to these bills, that a label or poster won't stop an alcoholic from drinking. Of course not. Nobody expects them to do so. The purpose of public education about drinking and pregnancy is to put into the common knowledge base of society the idea that a pregnant woman should not use alcohol. Just as everyone knows that overeating will make a person gain weight because it is "common knowledge," alcohol education will result in everyone knowing that alcohol harms the fetus, without having to go to special health classes or read articles on the subject.

Additional debate over warnings has centered around what message should be given to women about *abstinence* versus "light" or "occasional" drinking. As pointed out earlier, the data on fetal alcohol effects related to low quantities of alcohol intake is difficult to obtain and sometimes contradictory. The effects, so far as they are now known, may be subtle and relatively small in scale. Some have argued that recommending abstinence on the basis of such subtle effects will cause women who have been light drinkers before recognizing pregnancy to panic about possible harm to their unborn child and undergo unnecessary anxiety or even abortion.

As director of the New York State Division of Alcoholism and Alcohol Abuse from 1979 to 1983, I had a very personal responsibility in deciding how to advise the public. At the request of New York's Governor, I chaired a Fetal Alcohol Syndrome Prevention Task Force that recommended a state-wide education campaign. We had already experienced a public information campaign mounted by the alcoholic beverage industry (as an alternative to health warning labels) that avoided using the word "alcohol" entirely and mentioned only "excessive or abusive drinking" in pregnancy as a potential problem. As a government agency, we had to decide how to advise the women of New York.

My own conclusion, as expressed in a 1984 debate on the issue, is as follows:

> Because alcohol is not necessary to life or health during pregnancy, because there is reasonable evidence of harm, and because safe levels are not established, we should recommend non-drinking during pregnancy as the safest course. In doing so, we should be careful to state the basis upon which this recommendation is made, and not to exaggerate the risks of small amounts of alcohol. This has been done reasonably well in the public education materials advocating non-drinking during pregnancy that have had national

distribution. As research continues to elucidate the mechanism or mechanisms of alcohol's effects on the fetus, I believe that as responsible professionals we should advocate for a public policy that errs, if it must, on the side of safety. We cannot recommend, on the basis of present knowledge, that social drinking is harmless during pregnancy.

Professional Education

In addition to educating the public, preventing FAS/FAE requires all involved health professionals to understand current findings about drinking and pregnancy, to have sufficient training to recognize alcohol and other drug problems in their early stages in women, and to know how to refer these women effectively for treatment.

Several studies have evaluated the effectiveness of professional education programs related to FAS/FAE for health professionals. The New York State campaign was evaluated by Dr. Marcia Russell and colleagues at the New York State Research Institute on Alcoholism in Buffalo. They found that the information packages sent to all New York State obstetricians/gynecologists were read by 77 percent of their recipients and were generally found to be useful. As a group, these physicians were well informed about FAS, as indicated by response to a questionnaire on the subject. However, the data on their response to patients with drinking problems revealed that they referred far fewer cases than they identified.

A second study, performed by Dr. Ruth Little and colleagues in Seattle, looked at advice given by obstetricians before and after a FAS education program. After the program, more obstetricians inquired about alcohol use and recommended abstinence for their patients.

A third study, from Boston City Hospital, by Lyn Weiner and colleagues, explored the clinical behavior of obstetric residents who had been trained to be sensitive to drinking during pregnancy and to use a ten-question test (see page 37) to identify heavy drinkers. The drinking questionnaire was included in every chart, and the researchers monitored how often the resident or other members of the clinic staff administered it. When the study began, members of a research team were regularly present in the clinic, and the completion rate was 92 percent. However, after the researchers departed, the completion rate dropped progressively over the next two years to a low of 33 percent. This rate jumped back up to 59 percent after the department chairperson issued a directive on the subject and stressed the availability of consultation.

The results of the Boston City Hospital study illustrate the need for ongoing training, encouragement, and support to make professional education effective. Public policy can stimulate such education by requiring adequate screening of all obstetric patients in order to satisfy state or federal accreditation. So far, no such regulation has been implemented.

The Criminalization of Alcohol and Other Drug Use in Pregnancy

Until recently, public policies aimed at preventing FAS/FAE were all designed to improve the lot of women with alcohol and other drug problems, while preserving their individual rights and human dignity. However, there are other important and urgent policy issues currently under debate that pit the rights of the unborn fetus against those of the prospective mother who has chosen to bear the child. Although the "mother versus fetus" debate is most often framed in terms of compelling a pregnant woman to undergo Cesarean section or other medical treatment against her will for the sake of her fetus, the same principle (of prenatal child abuse) has been used to force pregnant women to abstain from alcohol and other drugs through threats of loss of custody or even incarceration. In addition, women have been prosecuted following childbirth for using alcohol or drugs during pregnancy.

In 1986, a California woman, whose premature infant died at age five days, allegedly because she took drugs while pregnant, was charged with criminal child neglect for not following medical advice during pregnancy. In another case, a Florida mother was convicted of the felony charge of delivering a controlled substance to a minor (cocaine metabolites through the umbilical cord, between the instant of birth and the severing of the cord). In *The Broken Cord*, Michael Dorris reported that on some American Indian reservations, jailing of pregnant women who would not (or could not) stop drinking has been recommended. This recommendation was made as a last resort by a community for whom both abortion and residential treatment are essentially unavailable.

Unavailability of services and the resulting frustration have given rise to a number of proposals to enforce abstinence from alcohol and other drugs or to prosecute women who do not abstain while pregnant. Proposed schemes have included mandatory treatment through the criminal justice system (with prison as an alternative if the patient fails to cooperate) and civil commitment to a treatment facility.

This trend seems to be the *least helpful* way to expend public funds for birth defect prevention. Forced "treatment" or jailing is being proposed for a population of women that has been offered neither humane and sensitive intervention nor access to culturally appropriate and effective treatment. As an example, the Florida woman mentioned above who was convicted of a felony had, in fact, contacted a drug hotline during her pregnancy, had expressed concern about her cocaine addiction, and had asked for help. She was told that no programs were available. When she went into labor, she also expressed her concern to her obstetrician. The result was that she was arrested postpartum, taken from the hospital in handcuffs, and prosecuted. The fact that her sentence included mandated treatment hardly seems to justify the way society responded to her need. The fact that she was poor and Black is also central to this trend. Both legal penalties for "prenatal child abuse" and urine drug testing and reporting of newborns tend to be applied to the disadvantaged in society—precisely those women who lack access to the help they need.

Penalties for pregnant women who use alcohol and other drugs or laws requiring mandatory reporting of pregnant addicts would have exactly the opposite results from those intended. Instead of improving the outcome of pregnancy, they would deter pregnant alcoholics and drug addicts from seeking help—both prenatal care and treatment for their chemical dependence. Fear of prosecution and incarceration is a strong motivator. If health professionals are mandated to report pregnant women who use alcohol or other drugs, they would be strongly motivated, but motivated to *avoid* recognizing the problem. Thus, punitive measures would work *against* every positive step taken by society to prevent FAS/FAE.

Rather than invest money in criminal justice approaches, we would do better to recognize the economic as well as the human benefits of rational FAS prevention.

Policy Recommendations

A full-scale FAS/FAE prevention policy should include:

1. Public education, including improved health warnings

2. Grade-appropriate school education at every level

3. Professional education for all health and human service professions

4. Systems to improve access to adequate prenatal care for all women

5. Systems to improve screening and referral for alcohol and drug problems in women in the health care system, especially obstetric care

6. Adequate, culturally sensitive, and accessible inpatient, residential, and outpatient chemical dependence treatment for every pregnant (and nonpregnant) woman in need

7. Vastly improved health, educational, and support systems to care for FAS/FAE-affected children

8. A community support system for parents and other caretakers of affected children

9. Additional research to improve our understanding of FAS/FAE and our ability to prevent and remediate its effect

This may sound like an ambitious and expensive program. However, undertaking such a program will be more economical in the long run than caring for the thousands of affected children born annually. We must make a choice. By not acting effectively, we also choose.

Health Questionnaire

The health questionnaire that follows is a self-test designed to be filled out by the patient in the waiting room. Alternatively, the questionnaire may be administered by a staff member. Its purpose is to alert the physician to possible alcohol problems and to the extent of self-reported smoking and alcohol use. It may also draw attention to the presence of emotional problems.

Please check answers below

1. When you are depressed or nervous, do you find any of the following helpful to feel better or to relax?

	VERY HELPFUL	NOT HELPFUL	NEVER TRIED
a. Smoking cigarettes	___	___	___
b. Working harder than usual at home or job	___	___	___
c. Taking a tranquilizer	___	___	___
d. Taking some other kind of pill or medication	___	___	___
e. Having a drink	___	___	___
f. Talking it over with friends or relatives	___	___	___

2. Think of the times you have been most depressed; at those times did you:

	YES	No
a. Lose or gain weight?	___	___
b. Lose interest in things that usually interest you?	___	___
c. Have spells when you couldn't seem to stop crying?	___	___
d. Suffer from insomnia?	___	___

3. Have you ever gone to a doctor, psychologist, social worker, counselor, or clergyman for help with an emotional problem?

YES	No
___	___

49

Please check one answer

4. How many cigarettes a day do you smoke?

    ___ More than 2 packs   ___ 1-2 packs

    ___ Less than 1 pack   ⌐ None

5. How often do you have a drink of wine, beer, or a beverage containing alcohol?

    ___ 3 or more times a day   ___ Once or twice a week

    ___ Twice a day   ___ Once or twice a month

    ___ Almost every day   ___ Less than once a month

                                           ___ Never

6a. If you drink wine, beer, or beverages containing alcohol, how often do you have four or more drinks in a day?

    ___ Almost always   ___ Frequently

    ___ Sometimes   ___ Never

6b. If you drink wine, beer or beverages containing alcohol, how often do you have one or two drinks in a day?

    ___ Almost always   ___ Frequently

    ___ Sometimes   ___ Never

7. What prescribed medications do you take?

    _____

    _____

    _____

8. What other drugs or medications do you use?

    _____

    _____

    _____

	YES	NO

9. Does your drinking or taking other drugs sometimes lead to problems between you and your family—that is, wife, husband, children, parent, or close relative?

10. During the past year, have close relatives or friends worried or complained about your drinking or taking other drugs?

11. Has a friend or family member ever told you about things while you were drinking or using other drugs that you do not remember?

12. Have you, within the past year, started to drink alcohol and found it difficult to stop before becoming intoxicated?

13. Has your father or mother ever had problems with alcohol or other drugs?

Evaluating the Health Questionnaire

Question   1   An answer of "very helpful" on c, d, or e should alert the physician to possible alcohol or drug dependence.

Questions 2 & 3   Any "yes" should alert the physician to possible emotional problems.

Questions   7-13   Any "yes" should alert the physician to possible alcohol problems.

Questions   4-6   Gives an indication of cigarette and alcohol use. Although patients with alcohol problems may under-report their drinking, the recorded data may be of considerable help.

If the physician suspects or is sure that the patient has a drinking problem:

1. Establish a firm diagnosis. Consult the *Diagnostic and Statistical Manual* (DSM) criteria for the diagnosis of alcoholism.

2. When consultation or referral is appropriate, consult or refer to:
    a.   a physician experienced in the treatment of alcoholism
    b.   an alcoholism treatment facility
    c.   your local council on alcoholism
    d.   Alcoholics Anonymous (listed in every telephone directory)

3. Refer family members and other concerned and interested persons close to the patient to:
    a.   a physician experienced in the treatment of alcoholism
    b.   an alcoholism treatment facility
    c.   your local council on alcoholism
    d.   Al-Anon family groups including Alateen for young family members (These groups may be contacted through telephone listings for Al-Anon or for Alcoholics Anonymous.)

Alternative Health Questionnaire

"TWEAK" Test

Do you drink alcoholic beverages? If you do, please take our "TWEAK" test.

T **Tolerance:** How many drinks does it take to make you feel high? *Record number of drinks at right.* ____

For the next questions, check "yes" or "no."

		YES	NO
W	Have close friends or relatives **Worried or Complained** about your drinking in the past year?	❑	❑
E	**Eye-Opener:** Do you sometimes take a drink in the morning when you first get up?	❑	❑
A	**Amnesia (Blackouts):** Has a friend or family member ever told you about things you said or did while you were drinking that you could not remember?	❑	❑
K(C)	Do you sometimes feel the need to **Cut Down** on your drinking?	❑	❑

To score the test, a seven-point scale is used. The tolerance question scores two points if a woman reports it takes two or more drinks for her to first begin to feel the effects of alcohol. (Think of the song "Tea for Two.") A positive response to the worry question scores two points. Each of the last three questions scores one point for positive responses. A total score of three or more points indicates the woman is likely to be a heavy/problem drinker.

For more information on screening, write to Marcia Russell, Ph.D., Research Institute on Alcoholism, 1021 Main Street, Buffalo, New York, 14203.

Reproduced with permission of Marcia Russell, Ph.D.

Recommended Readings

Entire Issue Devoted to Drinking and Pregnancy

Alcohol Alert, National Institute on Alcohol Abuse and Alcoholism, No. 13, PH 297, July 1991.

Alcohol Health & Research World, Vol. 10, No. 1, Fall 1985.

Alcoholism: Clinical and Experimental Research, Vol. 14, No. 5, October, 1990.

Sections of Special Reports to Congress Dealing with Drinking and Pregnancy

Alcohol and Health, Sixth Special Report to the U.S. Congress, pp. 80-96, January 1987.

Alcohol and Health, Seventh Special Report to the U.S. Congress, pp. 139-161, January 1990.

Books and Articles

Abel, Ernest L., et al. *Alcohol Syndrome and Fetal Alcohol Effects*, New York: Plenum, 1984.

Abel, Ernest L. and Robert J. Sokol, "A Revised Conservative Estimate of the Incidence of FAS and its Economic Impact." *Alcoholism, Clinical and Experimental Research*, Vol. 15, No. 3, June 1990, pp. 514-524.

Blume, Sheila B. *Alcohol/Drug Dependent Women: New Insights into Their Special Problems, Treatment, Recovery*. Minneapolis: Johnson Institute, 1988.

Blume, Sheila B. "Is Social Drinking During Pregnancy Harmless? There Is Reason to Think Not," paper presented at conference on Controversies in Alcoholism and Substance Abuse, sponsored by the National Association on Drug Abuse Problems, New York City, March 26, 1984. Also, published in *Advances in Alcohol & Substance Abuse*, Vol. 5, Nos. 1/2, 1986, pp. 209-219. Also in Stimmel, Barry (ed.), *Controversies in Alcoholism and Substance Abuse*, New York: Haworth Press, 1986, pp. 209-219.

Blume, Sheila B. "Women and Alcohol: A Review." *Journal of the American Medical Association,* Vol. 256, No. 11, Sept. 19, 1986, pp. 1467-1470.

Blume, Sheila B. "Women, Alcohol and Drugs," in Miller NS (ed.): *Comprehensive Handbook of Drug and Alcohol Addiction.* New York, Marcel Dekker, 1990, pp. 147-177.

Chavez, Gilberto F. "Leading Major Congenital Malformations Among Minority Groups in the United States," *Journal of the American Medical Association,* 1989, 261:205-209.

Chavkin, Wendy. "Mandatory Treatment for Drug Use During Pregnancy," *Journal of the American Medical Association* Vol. 266, No. 11, Sept. 18, 1991 pp. 1556-1561.

Clarren, Sterling. "Recognition of Fetal Alcohol Syndrome," *Journal of the American Medical Association,* Vol. 245, No. 23, June 19, 1981, pp. 2436-2439.

Dorris, Michael. *The Broken Cord.* New York: Harper & Row, 1989.

Ervin, Cynthia S., Ruth E. Little, and Ann P. Streissguth, et al. "Alcoholic Fathering and Its Relation to Child's Intellectual Development: A Pilot Investigation," *Alcoholism: Clinical and Experimental Research,* Vol. 8, No. 4, August 1984, pp. 362-365.

Ewing, John A. "Detecting Alcoholism: The CAGE Questionnaire," *Journal of the American Medical Association,* Vol. 252, No. 14, Oct. 12, 1984, pp. 1905-1907.

Halliday, Andrea, Booker Bush, Paul Cleary, et al. "Alcohol Abuse in Women Seeking Gynecologic Care," *Obstetrics & Gynecology,* Vol. 68, No. 3, September 1986 pp. 322-326.

Hoegerman, Georgeanne, Catherine Wilson, Ellen Thurmond, et al. "Drug-Exposed Neonates," *Western Journal of Medicine,* Vol. 152, No. 5, 1990, pp. 559-564.

Little, Ruth E., Kevin W. Anderson, Cynthia H. Ervin, et al. "Maternal Alcohol Use During Breast-Feeding and Infant Mental and Motor Development at One Year," *The New England Journal of Medicine,* Vol. 321, No. 7, August 17, 1989, pp. 425-430.

Little, Ruth E., Ann P. Streissguth, Gay M. Guzinski, et al. "Change in Obstetrician Advice Following a Two-Year Community Educational Program on Alcohol Use and Pregnancy," *American Journal of Obstetrics and Gynecology,* Vol. 146, No. 1, May 1, 1983, pp. 23-28.

Mills, James L., Barry I. Graubard, Earnest E. Harley, et al. "Maternal Alcohol Consumption and Birth Weight," *Journal of the American Medical Association,* Vol. 252, No. 14, October 12, 1984, pp. 1875-1879.

Office of Substance Abuse Prevention, *Prevention Resource Guide: Pregnant/Postpartum Women and Their Infants,* United States Dept. of Health and Human Services, June 1991.

Rodin, Alvin E. "Infants and Gin Mania in 18th-Century London," *Journal of the American Medical Association,* Vol. 245, No. 12, March 27, 1981.

Russell, Marcia. "Clinical Implications of Recent Research on the Fetal Alcohol Syndrome," *Bulletin of the New York Academy of Medicine,* 67:207-222, 1991.

Russell, Marcia and Jeremy B. Skinner. "Early Measures of Maternal Alcohol Misuse as Predictors of Adverse Pregnancy Outcomes," *Alcoholism: Clinical and Experimental Research,* Vol. 12, No. 6, December, 1988, pp. 824-830.

Russell, Marcia. "Screening for Alcohol Related Patients in Obstetric and Gynocologic Patients," in Abel, Ernest L. "Fetal Alcohol Syndrome," *Vol. II Human Studies,* Boca Raton, FL:CRC Press, Inc., 1982, pp. 1-19.

Smith, Iris E., Juliana S. Lancaster, Suzette Moss-Wells, et al. "Identifying High-Risk Pregnant Drinkers: Biological and Behavioral Correlates of Continuous Heavy Drinking during Pregnancy," *Journal of Studies on Alcohol,* Vol. 48, No. 4, 1987, pp. 304-309.

Sokol, Robert J., Susan S. Martier, and Joel W. Ager. "The T-ACE Questions: Practical Prenatal Detection of Risk-drinking," *American Journal of Obstetrics and Gynecology,* Vol. 160, No. 4, April 1989, pp. 863-870.

Streissguth, Ann P. "What Every Community Should Know About Drinking During Pregnancy and the Lifelong Consequences for Society," The 1990 Betty Ford Lecture, in *Substance Abuse,* Vol. 12, No. 3, 1991, pp. 114-127.

Streissguth, Ann P., Jon M. Aase, Sterling K. Clarren, et al. "Fetal Alcohol Syndrome in Adolescents and Adults," *Journal of the American Medical Association,* Vol. 265, No. 15, April 17, 1990, pp. 1961-1967.

Streissguth, Ann P., Sharon Landesman-Dwyer, Joan C. Martin, et al. "Teratogenic Effects of Alcohol in Humans and Laboratory Animals," *Science,* Vol. 209, July 18, 1980, pp. 353-361.

United States Department of Health and Human Services. *A Manual on Adolescents and Adults with Fetal Alcohol Syndrome with Special Reference to American Indians.* Indian Health Services, 1986.

Warner, Rebecca H. and Henry L. Rosett. "The Effects of Drinking on Offspring: An Historical Survey of the American and British Literature," *Journal of Studies on Alcohol,* Vol. 36, No. 11, 1975, pp. 1395-1420.

Weiner, Lyn, Henry L. Rosett, and Kenneth C. Edelin. "Behavioral Evaluation of Fetal Alcohol Education for Physicians," *Alcoholism: Clinical and Experimental Research,* Vol. 6, No. 2, Spring 1982, pp. 230-233.

Recommended Reading for Patients and Family Members

Barry Robe, Lucy. *Just So It's Healthy.* Minneapolis: CompCare Publications, 1982.

Barry Robe, Lucy. *Alcohol and Pregnancy: Why They Don't Mix.* Chicago: American Medical Association, 1984.

National Institute on Alcohol Abuse and Alcoholism. *My Baby: Strong and Healthy.* United States Department of Health and Human Services, No. ADM86-1436, 1986.

Office of Substance Abuse Prevention. *How to Take Care of Your Baby Before Birth.* United States Department of Health and Human Services, No. ADM91-1557, 1991.

32-IQ

Cheese pizza